FRONT COVER illustration by Marshall Ramsey of Madison, Mississippi, twice nominated for the Pulitzer Prize and syndicated editorial cartoonist for the Jackson, Mississippi, *Clarion-Ledger* newspaper.

CHARCOAL DRAWING of author by nationally award-winning pastel artist, Cecilia Edgeworth Baker of Ridgeland, Mississippi.

# Hot Flashes, Swollen Ankles and Sore Breasts. And I'm a Man.

## How One Man Used a Sense of Humor to Combat Cancer - Twice

Bob Vance Moulder

authorHOUSE®

AuthorHouse™
1663 Liberty Drive
Bloomington, IN 47403
www.authorhouse.com
Phone: 1-800-839-8640

First published by AuthorHouse   8/7/2009

ISBN: 978-1-4490-0160-5 (e)
ISBN: 978-1-4490-0159-9 (sc)

Printed in the United States of America
Bloomington, Indiana

This book is printed on acid-free paper.

# Dedication

To Jerry Moulder, a very special brother.
And  to the memory of  John "Duke" Wayne - actor,
humanitarian, patriot - a man of strength, courage
and honor  in every sense of the words.

# A Pledge

I pledge ten percent of any personal profits
derived from the sale of this book to
the John Wayne Cancer Foundation.

*"Courage is being
scared to death - but
saddling up anyway."*
*- John Wayne*

# A Special Thanks

To the devoted radiation staff at the
St. Dominic Cancer Center: Alice, Amy,
Arnetter, Bryan, Crissy, Dale, Dianne,
Emily, Jennifer, Lois, Marcus, M.J., Peggy,
Stephanie, and Suzanne.
Professionals all.  Friends forever.

# Introduction

The three most caring and soul-stirring words in any language are "I love you." I know. I have spoken the words many times to my family and to my many concerned friends. I've also been fortunate to have heard the words from the same wonderful people.

On the other side of the verbal coin, the three most frightening, the most dreaded, the most gut-wrenching words ever heard are, "You have cancer," when spoken by a physician.

I am also familiar with those words. I've experienced the shock, the pain, and the feeling of terror that instantly erased every other thought from my mind except for the nagging dread of impending death.

I heard the words, "You have cancer," spoken to my father who had prostate cancer in his late seventies. I heard them spoken to my mother who died of an inoperable brain tumor, to my wife who faced the trauma of cancer in both lungs and died at the young age of 63, and to my younger brother who is now undergoing treatment for cancer in both lungs.

I heard them spoken to me in 2004 by my urologist when a biopsy confirmed I had prostate cancer, and I heard them spoken again to me in early 2009 when a pathology report determined an obstruction on my right lung at the end of my bronchial tube contained cancer cells.

Having heard the dreaded words so many times, I was much more prepared when they were spoken to me in 2009.

This time I was not afraid and I did not feel sorry for myself.

I was angry.

In the language of my Mississippi redneck brothers, "I was just flat pissed off."

I made up my mind before I left the doctor's office that I would face this battle as I had with every other problem in my life - head on.

As I told my physician when she, hesitantly, broke the news to me, "Look Doctor, you're not talking to a whiner here. Let's get it on. Let's do whatever needs to be done to eliminate that sucker from my body."

There are two ways you can handle hearing the words, "You have cancer."

You can break down and cry, moan and groan, gnash your teeth, cover yourself with sackcloth and ashes, feel sorry for yourself, cast blame on everyone and everything for your problems, and retreat into a shell of your own making; wasting precious days, weeks, months or possibly years of the time granted to you on this beautiful green planet.

Or you can get mad as hell and vow you will not be intimidated.

You can kick butts and take names, fight with every source at your command, and rather than living in terror, you can live to the fullest every day God grants you as a blessing, and view the entire process with a sense of humor, faith and a positive attitude.

As for me, I have chosen to fight. And when I say fight, I don't mean a *political correctness* slap on the face. I mean fight tooth and talon, no holds barred, claws and fangs.

There are no genes in my mental or physical makeup that will allow me to shrink into a corner and give up. And when I fight, I always do it with the full expectations of winning.

Yet if death is to be my final destiny in this battle, then let it be known that I fought every step of the way. I never backed down. I neither accepted defeat, nor did I allow the almost insurmountable odds of survival to dissuade me.

Let it be remembered that I faced my enemy with the same true grit shown by 300 brave Spartans who died side-by-side at the battle of Thermopylae; a battle they knew in the long run they could not win against millions of Persian invaders, yet a battle they had no choice but to fight if they were to continue thinking of themselves as men and as warriors.

In my initial prayer after my cancer was diagnosed, both in 2004 and 2009, I said, "God I'm placing myself in your hands. This does not mean I'm not going to fight this insidious parasite for as long as I have the strength, in every avenue open to me. But after all is said and done, what happens to me is Your choice, Your plan, and I'll accept Your verdict."

# 1

**I** have always had a weird sense of humor. I have also been blessed with a vivid imagination; the ability to find something unique, unusual and most of the time funny out of dire situations.

For me, imagination has meant the difference between following an ill-tempered mule up and down red clay cotton rows in south Mississippi where I was born and raised, or filming pretty girls on Brazil's Copacabana beach with the benefit of a liberal expense account.

It has meant the difference between writing my stories in an air-conditioned office, or crawling out of bed before daylight to feed the chickens, slop the hogs and milk uncooperative cows that never enjoyed the feel of my cold hands.

Imagination has made it possible for me to travel throughout much of the world rather than simply reading about far-off places in newspapers and magazines.

More importantly, since I was diagnosed with prostate cancer in 2004 and had to undergo radiation treatments every day for eight weeks, my imagination enabled me to survive in a fantasy world rather than dwelling on the reality of what was actually happening to my body.

Every day when I stretched out on a hard table and prepared myself for the "zapping" I knew was coming, I invented stories I knew were not true, but never-the-less stories that made the routine of my treatment far more bearable.

I pictured myself taking a twilight stroll in my nice middle-class neighborhood, enjoying the coolness of twilight, when suddenly garage doors started opening and closing with rapidity.

Microwave ovens turned on and off, porch lights blinked with the regularity of Christmas tree decorations, and irate neighbors screamed at me to go home and put on a protective lead overcoat so all the radiation in my body would not contaminate the neighborhood.

I imagined commercial and military jets cruising peacefully on auto-pilot at 38,000 feet until they passed directly over me and began performing uncontrollable barrel rolls, figure eights and loops.

I visualized the expressions of Shopping Mall security guards when anti-theft devices set off car horns all over the parking lot when I got out of my lead-lined vehicle to go inside to shop; and people wearing hearing aids grabbing their ears and screaming in agony when I moved within their range.

I'm sure many of you think a man of my age fantasizing about such things while undergoing a serious procedure like radiation for an even more serious disease like cancer is rather ridiculous - perhaps, even a bit silly.

But my imagination has been a salvation for me during hard and trying times since I was a small boy growing up on a 40-acre-and-a-mule farm during the Great Depression.

My fantasies were all I had to occupy my time.

I remember distinctly when I began creating the imaginary images that would later enable me to survive diversity when it would have been so easy to give in to the pressures and feel sorry for myself.

I sat cross-legged on the front porch of our faded, rough-lumber farm house and listened in total rapture as an old hobo reminisced about his life on the road.

Every gesture the tattered old man made with crusty, arthritic hands massaged my imagination. Each word he spoke nourished my dreams.

Fueled by his often exaggerated tales, my imagination took flight. It introduced me to a wondrous life that existed outside the red clay hills of south Mississippi.

While the old hobo sipped from a dipper of cool well water, I closed my eyes, trying to visualize all the exciting places he had talked about.

The old man patted me on the head. "You're alright, boy. You like hearing me talk about all the places I've been, don't you?"

"Yes, sir, and someday I'm gonna do the same thing."

"How old are you, boy?"

"Tomorrow's my birthday. I'll be ten-years-old."

"That's what I figured. Still, you're about the age I was when I caught my first freight out of Oklahoma." He paused a second. "I'll be leaving directly - if you want to tag along. We'll head down the road until we hit the big water. Then we'll flip a coin and put our trust in lady luck. Well, boy, you want to go with me?"

As young as I was, I knew the old man had no intentions of taking me with him. I also knew I wouldn't get ten feet from the house before my father grabbed me by the nape of the neck and turned me over his knee. But I wanted to go. I wanted to go so badly I could feel the bottoms of my bare feet tingling.

I envied the free-wheeling hobos. But I didn't envy them enough, or want to go badly enough, to accept the hunger, the deprivation or the loss of pride they endured to maintain their chosen lifestyle.

The Depression had taught me what doing without was like. It also taught me how to recognize God-given talents - my imagination, sense of humor and a positive attitude - that would in the future make my life bearable; both emotionally and financially.

When my parents decided to bring me into their world, they earned a respectable living teaching at eighth grade rural schools during the winter and working a 40-acre farm during the summer.

The three-room house, where we camped during the summer between school sessions, had no insulation in the walls or flooring. Where there should have been a ceiling, 2"x4" rafters spaced 24 inches apart crossed each room eight feet above the floor.

The last thing I saw every night before turning out the lamp, and the first thing I saw every morning when I opened my eyes, were those bare rafters above my head.

With one exception.

Early one spring morning during my sixth year, I awoke staring into the slitted eyes of a five-foot-long rattlesnake coiled around a rafter directly above my head.

Its triangular head hung down about six inches.

Its forked tongue flitted in and out so rapidly each movement blurred into the other.

I was hypnotized, unable to move.

Screams built inside my chest, but I heard no sound. When a mournful whimper finally broke through my terror, it led the way for screams that literally blasted my parents up from the breakfast table.

Seeing me sitting up in bed with my eyes locked on the rattlesnake slowly descending from the rafter, my father reacted without thinking.

He grabbed a single-barrel, .410 gauge shotgun he kept beside his bed, pointed at the snake and pulled the trigger.

The load of birdshot blasted a hole in the cedar-shingle roof the size of a basketball.

Wood splinters, accumulated dirt dauber nests and several bloody pieces of a still-writhing rattlesnake splattered the clean, sun-dried sheets mother had put on the bed the night before.

Pieces of the rattler's body barely touched me before she jerked me out of bed like a field worker handling a 100-pound sack of fertilizer.

The next morning, dad rewarded me with a rare 5-cent candy bar for my bravery by taking me to Mr. George's Store, the one-and-only shopping emporium in the tiny rural community of Lorena where we lived.

In fact, you might say the store was Lorena if you discounted the gristmill, a dilapidated wooden building slowly settling under its own weight, and my preacher grandfather's house, a six-room dogtrot structure located diagonally across the narrow dirt road from the store.

Yet it was around Mr. George's store that life revolved in the community.

The narrow, ship-lap, frame building with its doublewide, unscreened front door, potbelly stove, manually operated gasoline pump, and outdoor ice box large as a bathroom in many of today's homes, was also Lorena's town hall.

It was a meeting place where farmers, loafers, and unemployed farm hands gathered to sit around the stove and swap stories. Since television did not exist and there were few battery radios in the community in the early 1930's, the store was also a place to hear travelers relate news of the world outside the borders of our tiny community.

Everybody in a ten-mile circle bought, sold, or traded with Mr. George at one time or the other. So he knew most of their secrets. But the regular loafers at the store knew that whatever secrets Mr. George knew, he would never reveal to anyone else. They just pointed at a sign hanging over the door: ***"Keep Your Mouth Shut, Your Bowels Open, and Believe in Jesus."***

Before my father and I arrived at the store that morning, I agonized over what I would buy with my nickel. Would I buy a Baby Ruth candy bar, or perhaps twenty-five foil-wrapped chocolate kisses? Or would I buy a Coca-Cola or a peach soda? Maybe I would torture myself by buying an Orange Crush in a brown bottle that didn't allow me to see how much was left until the last drop was gone.

Between the kidding I received from the store loafers who wanted to advise me how to spend my nickel, and the indecision I went through staring into showcases and drink boxes, it took a long ten minutes to decide on my special treat.

After joking with me for several minutes, and making suggestions as to what I should buy, the loafers became so interested in their argument over what I should buy, they forgot I was there.

I was pleased. I could take all the time I needed to make up my mind.

Eating only a nibble of candy at a time, or sipping just enough of my drink to wet the inside of my mouth, I managed to extend my pleasures.

Sitting cross-legged on the counter where Mr. George measured yards of cloth from colorful bolts Mother could rarely afford, I drank in their yarns with every sip of soda and with every bite of already melting candy that clung to the roof of my mouth like sweet glue.

Even though there was little I enjoyed more than listening while a group of old men sat around a pot-bellied stove in the store and told stories, I was never allowed to participate. But on that never-to-be-forgotten Saturday, my Uncle "Cutthroat" Jim surprised me by saying, "Take the floor, boy. It's all yours. Let's hear about your snake."

For close to an hour, surrounded by masters of the storytelling art, I stretched, grimaced and enlarged on a tale destined to become a classic whenever and wherever men gathered to chew, spit and swap tall tales. And my father earned the dubious reputation as being the only man in south Mississippi to blow a hole in the ceiling of his house while in the process of killing a rattlesnake.

I realized that day if I could make a living telling stories, if I could utilize my sense of humor and could allow the fantasies created by my imagination to be released unabated, my life would be far more enjoyable than following an ill-tempered mule up and down a cotton row.

That is what I have done for more than fifty years. My life has not only been enjoyable, but my stories have also been profitable enough for me to support my family in a much better manner than if I had I remained at home and became a farmer.

Many people, even some of my close friends, cannot understand how I can make jokes when I am drowning in sorrow or worries. But those are the times when humor tosses me a life preserver and brings me back to solid ground.

While sitting in a cancer center lobby with nearly a dozen other patients waiting my turn to be treated with radiation, I jokingly told a man sitting beside me that so many members of my family had suffered from cancer that when we planned a family reunion the first invitations we mailed went to various cancer societies and foundations.

The majority, who overheard my statement, understood and apparently appreciated my sense of humor. But one woman, unattractive at her best, apparently was in the minority.

Sitting across from me with her hands gripping the chair handles as if she unclenched them God would surely snatch her away in a cloud of radioactive dust, she obviously took umbrage at my discussing cancer in such a lighthearted manner.

"You should be ashamed making jokes about something as terrible as," and she whispered the word, "cancer. Don't you realize all these people are terrified of dying from," and again she whispered, "cancer" almost as if she said the word aloud the angel of death would strike her down without the opportunity to make even one last wish.

I thought of many ways to answer her question - and some would have filled me with a perverse satisfaction. But none were befitting of the training I had received from a doting mother and grandmother about how to conduct myself as a true southern gentleman.

Fortunately, I was saved from what could have been an embarrassing altercation when her name was called. She paused a moment at the doorway to the radiation chamber to glare at me one last time as if confirming her opinion of me was lower than dirt.

I'm not sure what I would have said to her if she had remained, but I like to think I would have told her more people have survived cancer with faith, humor and a positive attitude than have ever been cured by burying their heads in the sand.

# 2

After my wife of more than four decades was diagnosed with lung cancer in 1987, I went through all the feelings that go with such a diagnosis; disbelief, anger, and finally just plain numbness.

When her oncologist told her she had a maximum of six months to live, she bowed her back and said, "No way will I die before my grandson is born."

She went through two painful surgeries, a long bout with chemo and eight weeks of radiation, yet she lived not six months as predicted, but six years. And she flew from Mississippi to Minnesota and held her grandson in her arms only minutes after he was born.

During those six years, I retired early and we did all the things we had dreamed of doing after I retired.

We spent almost a month with our daughter, an army officer and helicopter pilot stationed in the Bavarian part of Germany. During that Christmas month, we traveled over much of snow-covered Germany, Austria and Switzerland. We spent two weeks in the Caribbean on the beautiful island of St. John, and finally we took a two-month driving tour through the American West.

Those are the beautiful memories I have retained, not the painful ones. There were other memories that will always be with me and are helping me to endure my own cancer treatment; her strength, her sense of humor, her faith and her positive attitude.

When she died six years after her original diagnosis, two months before my 65th birthday, I was lost.

It would have taken so little effort for me to lean back in my rocking chair and succumb to the slow, boring existence that befalls many people after retirement - especially after the loss of a spouse.

But I didn't.

I fought with everything I had not to give in either to age or to my grief. I was resolved not to sit at home and feel sorry for myself.

I was equally determined to find the will and the strength to abandon my fears, to find out the difference between just surviving and really living during my so-called golden years.

Still, my fight was not easy. I went through many trying times, many painful times, and many long days and even longer nights.

Then I remembered something my wife said to me not long before she died. "I want your promise that you won't give up when I'm gone," she said. "I want your word you won't waste your life sitting at home grieving. I want you to live, to see this country as we have planned for so many years."

I nodded, but I promptly erased the idea from my mind. Traveling alone was a problem I didn't want to face, to even think about. Yet in my grief, I finally realized with a clarity I had not experienced since her death she was right as usual, that perhaps traveling alone was something I should consider.

Since I had traveled throughout this country and much of the world during my work years, and since those years had been spent as a writer, I asked myself - what better way than travel and writing about my travels to ease my pain and to find myself again?

I had to create a new life, and exercising the vagabond dreams of my childhood to follow the sun was the most logical solution I had yet found.

A few weeks later, after buying a small fifth-wheel trailer and the biggest, blackest, longest, tallest, most intimidating, Bubba-bragging, bad-assed pickup on the lot at my local Chevrolet dealership, I abandoned the long-standing security of home, family, friends and – equally as important – routine, in order to follow an endless highway with nothing but a life-long dream to guide me and a newly discovered courage to push me.

No itinerary.

No destination other than a far-distant horizon and the wonders of God's beautiful green earth unfolding through my windshield.

That's what I did for eight years, and not a single day did I regret my decision.

During one of my rare trips back home, I reluctantly made an appointment with my physician for a physical examination.

The doctor caught me by surprise toward the end with three words: "Bend over," and "Gotcha." The following day he called me with news he was making an appointment for me with a urologist.

When I asked why, he said, "Your prostate is abnormally large, your records show your father had prostate cancer, the disease is hereditary, and your tests show your PSA blood test is several points higher than the norm. Any other questions?"

For macho-type men who show off among their friends by beating on their chests like a mountain gorilla during the mating season, the idea of going into a urologist's office for a prostate exam is somewhat akin to a 375-pound defensive tackle attending a cross-dresser's ball wearing nothing but a powder blue camisole.

How do I know? It takes one to catch one.

For years I put off having the testing because the idea of another man examining me in the undignified way a prostate exam has to be done was too abhorrent to even contemplate.

My first visit resulted in me being tested every six months for more than ten years, enduring three biopsies which felt very much like someone had wrapped a rough oak 4x4 with a live 220 wire and stuffed the entire post, splinters and all - well, I won't go any further with my description since I'm sure you get the picture.

Following the final biopsy, my urologist called a halt to my traveling when he dropped the frightening "cancer" word on me.

Even though I thought I had prepared myself for positive results during all the years of testing, the second my doctor confirmed my cancer, I reacted as any normal person would react: shortness of breath that felt like I had run six marathons across Kenya, a dry mouth and a heart that pounded like a bass drum inside my chest.

Like everyone else who has been told he or she has cancer, I was not ready. I had always naively thought it would be to someone else. Certainly it would never happen to me

My doctor followed up by saying since I had been tested twice a year for almost a decade, the cancer was in its beginning stages and was still confined within the prostate.

He assured me with proper treatment, combined with a lot of luck, a positive attitude, and, he stressed, a sense of humor, my cancer was curable.

As TV's Maverick once said when he was called a coward because he wouldn't leave a card game to face down a drunk in the street "A hero dies only once but a coward dies a thousand deaths. I like them odds."

I liked my odds and I refused to entertain or accept any other thought but a complete cure.

Since I have always believed that knowledge is power, I tried to learn everything I could about my enemy, its weaknesses and how it could be defeated. Then I met it in open field combat swinging with all my might.

Paraphrasing a Chinese general named Sun Tzu, who more than 2,000 years ago wrote, *The Art of War,* "If you know your enemies then you will be able to attack them . . . but the individual, without strategy, who takes his opponent lightly, will immediately become a captive."

The main thing I discovered about having cancer was I could not - and would not - go around whining and feeling sorry for myself. I had to face my trials with confidence, with faith, and with my own quirky sense of humor that is often misunderstood and occasionally not appreciated.

# 3

During my preliminary tests and subsequent treatments for prostate cancer, I found for some unexplainable reason when a man whose body is in his early eighties – but his mind still thinks he is in his mid-40's where women are concerned – the females who examine or treat him are invariably attractive, shapely, and not a day older than 30.

They are usually blond, have a slight overbite that emphasizes full, pouty lips, and invariably, they emit just a hint of perfume when they get close enough to cause an old man like me to undergo unforgettable indignities during their examinations.

During my initial battle with prostate cancer in 2004, I thought it was purely coincidental that both my radiologist and oncologist had hired attractive young women as their assistants. But during my recent bout with lung cancer, I came to the conclusion it was not coincidence.

It was a carefully and diabolically conceived plan on the part of physicians to find out if their aged male patients still had enough life left for them to bother with trying to get them on their feet again.

Yet I could not help but think there also might be another reason - a divine reason.

Each time I was either examined or treated, and looked into a mirror to see a gray-haired, pot-bellied man in his early eighties staring back at me, I had to believe having beautiful young women treat me was part of an overall master plan of punishment for my misspent youth.

Another indignity for a knobby-kneed old man like me to suffer was being forced to wear a gown that exposed more of my body than few people, other than my mother and wife, had ever seen.

You know the kind.

Your front side is covered, but your entire backside is exposed for the entire world to see.

To make it even worse, my wife and mother only saw the outside of my body.

With the use of computers, monitors, probes and other technology a novice like me could only imagine, the health care professionals could also see my insides – which probably was even less exciting to a young woman than my outside sags and wrinkles.

The first time I experienced such an indignity was during my first prostate biopsy.

I was sent into a tiny room by an attractive nurse who instructed me to take off all my clothing and to slip into the gown in preparation for the biopsy.

A few minutes later, she knocked on the door to find me backed into a corner with my left hand behind me gripping the open part of my gown. She led me into another room and told me to stretch out on the table with my rear end facing her and to assume the fetal position.

Trying to obey her orders while keeping my modesty was no easy job.

When I finally managed to assume the position she demanded, she laughed. "Why are you trying so hard to keep your rear end covered? I've probably seen more men's behinds while working in this job than you have seen throughout your life. Believe me, on a scale of one to ten, your little flat butt is not so special you would make such an effort to keep it covered."

I had always known that my butt was flat, possibly even inverted. There has never been anything about my behind that has caused women to pause and whistle when I walk past them on the street. But to be told by an attractive woman that my behind was nothing to be proud of was an embarrassment, and frankly an insult.

When the nurse left the room and the doctor entered, I was vastly relieved until I saw him holding a tray with six needles as long as my forearm.

I became frantic.

"Doctor, I've heard of the Chinese using acupuncture to cure certain diseases, but those needles are ridiculous."

He laughed. "We are going to use a probe with a light and camera on the end to record photos of your prostate on a television monitor."

"A probe? Are you saying what I think you're saying?"

He laughed again. For some reason my imagination conceived a picture of a medieval torturer turning the rack one more notch on some poor serf who had already been stretched four inches taller.

"The probe has a tiny hole through the center where I insert one of these needles," he explained, "and remove a bite of your prostate for later analysis. Don't worry, it's not that painful."

I thought again about the man on the torture rack.

I was feeling bad enough at the thought of having one of those long needles inserted into my body, when the door opened and the attractive nurse I thought had left for the day entered the room with what the doctor called a "probe" held in her hands.

My immediate thought when I saw it was remembering a cattle prod I once used to help my grandfather herd his cows into a pen.

Only larger.

"What is she doing here?" I asked, even though I had a sickening feeling I knew.

"I can't probe and take biopsies at the same time," he said with a mischievous smile.

At that point I had no choice but to close my eyes, grip the bed frame with both hands, and endure each snip that felt very much like I imagined it would feel when the Gestapo used pliers to pull out prisoners' fingernails in an effort to make them talk.

When I related my feelings about the Gestapo to my urologist, he accepted his role with gusto.

"Get ready," he said as he inserted the first needle, "here comes the little fingernail. Now here is the middle finger - the thumb." Suddenly my feeble attempt at humor was no longer funny.

Except to him.

During all the tests and treatments I endured, another question I had always wanted to ask crossed my mind.

I had been under the impression that doctors and other medical personnel used alcohol to sterilize their instruments and their hands. If that premise is true, I wondered, why do they have to keep both in a freezer prior to using them on a patient?

To be honest, I'm sure they don't really keep their instruments in a freezer. But each time I wore one of those backless gowns and a doctor touched my bare skin with a stethoscope, the chill bumps that popped up on my body was evidence enough for me to believe doctors keep their instruments cold on purpose in order to jump start a patient's bodily functions.

Have you ever stretched out on a table in a hospital or clinic where they keep the temperature cold enough to store meat; especially wearing a backless gown? It feels akin to sliding on your back down a snow bank - naked.

During my first visit to the Cancer Center to began my eight long weeks of radiation, which would turn out to be every day except weekends, I was ushered down a long, antiseptically scrubbed hallway for a CAT scan; a hallway I guessed would look and smell like the customer waiting room at a Dr. Tischner's Antiseptic manufacturing plant.

Being somewhat claustrophobic - no, a lot claustrophobic would be more descriptive - I pictured myself being rolled into a huge tube reminiscent of the old iron lungs people of my generation saw almost every time a newsreel appeared at a movie theater during the 1940's.

By that time my churning stomach was bouncing up and down like a bowling ball on a trampoline.

When we entered the room where the "scanner" was located, I realized the mistake I had made comparing it to an iron lung - as well as allowing myself to succumb to claustrophobia unnecessarily.

At first glance, the scanner reminded me of a clothes washer, with neither a top nor a bottom, lying on its side on top of a long, hard, and, I correctly assumed, uncomfortable table.

Once I stretched out, with the exception of the table being cool to my bare bottom, there was nothing about the scan that was either painful or claustrophobic.

The washing machine, as I affectionately called the scanner, never covered my entire body at one time. True, my body passed through its circular confines, but only an inch or so at a time, never enough for me to feel the least bit claustrophobic.

Since I was told the procedure would last 20 or so minutes, I closed my eyes and started to compare myself to a load of clothing. At first, since I was calm and relatively comfortable, I figured I was in the *Wash Cycle*.

The scanner moved very slowly over my body, taking what seemed to me like hundreds of individual pictures.

Every time the scanner moved a fraction of an inch or so, its motor groaning and rattling like an old washing machine with a crank wringer we used to own, the block under my head - that looked very much like the block my father, the mortician, used when he was embalming a body - became less and less comfortable.

I started to notice things I had not paid any attention to in the beginning; the rubber ring holding my feet together so I could not move, another rubber ring I gripped with each hand so my arms would remain stationary, how hard the table was under my bony shoulders.

I figured I had finally progressed to the *Rinse Cycle*.

Seconds later, the sound and movement stopped and the therapist moved the scanner away from my body and helped me sit up. I had been so involved in my imaginary washing cycles, my skin actually felt damp when a cool blast from the overhead air conditioning unit hit me.

It was not until I stepped out of the building into the warmth of a Mississippi summer day, that I finally felt like the scan I had been unnecessarily dreading was over.

I was now in my *Drying Cycle,* and heading toward home where I planned to *fold* into my easy chair with a sun-*Downy* or two - oops, meant to say a sundowner - *press* my head into a soft pillow, and *hang* the world out to *dry.*

*"When you come slam
bang up against trouble,
it never looks half as bad
if you face up to it."*

*John Wayne*

# 4

One of the most awkward embarrassments I had to face during my long weeks of radiation treatment was standing in front of a mirror attempting to bathe my body with a Q-Tip.

I suppose bathing with a Q-tip is somewhat of an exaggeration.

Yet when almost a third of my body was covered with a multitude of black permanent markers that resembled ancient Egyptian hieroglyphics I had been ordered not to remove - either by one of my honey-voiced female therapists or one of the three male therapists who might be walk-on's at a New Orleans Saints training camp - I took all measures to do as I was told.

While looking into a mirror and trying to negotiate a zig-zag path between all the black marks like a laboratory rat trying to find its way through a maze, my overall cleanliness depended either on a package of Q-tips or my dexterity with the tip of a bath cloth.

Without access to a seamstress who could provide me with a pair of waterproof plastic bloomers large enough to cover the lower part of my torso, enjoying a tub bath or a shower was virtually impossible.

At the time, a long, cold shower would truly have been delightful.

Please don't laugh when I tell you that prior to my radiation treatments, I suffered terribly from PMS.

No, not the kind you're thinking about. My PMS, which I called *Post Macho Syndrome*, began when my urologist put me on a 16-month-long hormone regimen.

It was bad enough for me to walk among young, attractive and shapely women and know the hormone shots had depleted not only all my testosterone, but also any - well, most thoughts of a sexual nature.

It was even worse living with an embarrassing malady I never dreamed a man would have to endure.

*Hot Flashes.*

Yes, I said, hot flashes.

Now, ladies, you may take a small intermission to giggle just a little, perhaps even to gloat.

And why not?

You certainly wouldn't be the only ones to find humor in my unusual misfortune.

I found out quickly that the female species has no sympathy for a man suffering from such an unusual malady.

Every woman I have told over the years seemed to enjoy a sadistic satisfaction that a man suffered from the same painful malady women have endured since Eve searched vainly throughout the tropical Garden of Eden for an ice bag to put on the back of her neck.

I think when God created women with menopausal hot flashes, He must have anticipated men would make crude jokes and laugh at their agony.

In my humble opinion, that's why He stuck us with an exclusive and worrisome body part called a prostate gland - an act I call anticipated punishment.

I shall never forget the time I took an attractive middle-age lady to dinner at an elegant restaurant and was joined by a mixed group of friends.

During the dinner my companion, a buxom lady who happened to be wearing a low-neck, scoop blouse that kept my mind off of my meal throughout the evening, was also suffering from periodic hot flashes.

Unaware of what she was doing, she kept lowering her head and blowing her breath down her blouse in a vain attempt to find relief.

One of the men leaned over and said, "I have seen women blow on their food, I've seen women blow on their coffee, and I've even seen women blow in their date's ear, but I don't think I've ever dined before with a woman who blew on her breasts."

The comment, which led to loud laughter from the men - including me - brought instant, squint-eyed silence from the women who knew the source of her problem.

That incident was a part of my life BC – *Before Cancer* - before my urologist decided to treat me with hormones rather than surgery.

His first thought was to use the radiation seeds, but my prostate was too large. The purpose of the hormone shots, even though they didn't work as he had hoped, was to hopefully shrink the prostate.

Before I left his office that morning, a tough acting nurse with a Marine drill sergeant mindset, ordered me to drop my pants. Then she popped me in the behind with a shot I later learned cost a great deal more money than my first new automobile.

Not long after I received the shot, the hot flashes began – slowly and deceptively gentle at first. Then they hit me with a vengeance.

I would be sitting still, perfectly comfortable, when suddenly, like a volcano building heat from inside a crater and then erupting in a cloud of smoke and ash, sweat would explode from thousands of pores on my face and chest.

Not having been prepared from childhood for such a calamitous occurrence, as women have been through the ages by their mothers, I immediately called my physician's office.

I was told by a syrupy voiced nurse, "Hot flashes are normal with hormone injections. But there is a medication that will help if you want a prescription."

"Naaaaaa," I said, still attempting to be macho.

"Then you'll just have to – hehehe – live with it," she giggled.

After four months of suffering, particularly at night when I would wake up with my body covered with sweat and throw off my covers, then wake up again with a chill when a blast of air conditioning hit me, I finally relented and asked for help.

To put the finishing touches on my embarrassment, when I took my prescription to the pharmacist, I told the young woman behind the counter I would wait for it to be filled.

Later, she said in a voice reminiscent of Mother Teresa, but one that could be heard throughout the length and breadth of the waiting area, "Mr. Moulder, your prescription for hot flashes is ready."

To add insult to injury while I gave her my insurance card and finally walked red-faced through a waiting room filled with grinning women, I glanced at the bold print on my prescription bottle. It read: **For Hot Flashes.**

"Lord," I whispered, "if you will help me get through this ordeal, if you will make sure this prescription works, I will never make fun of women again."

I have always believed the God I worship has a sense of humor; a belief that is justified every time I look into a mirror. To a certain extent He proved it that day.

The prescription worked immediately and the hot flashes slowed almost to a stop. But just to keep me from getting cocky about Him answering my prayer, He replaced my hot flashes with swollen ankles and sore boobs.

I know you have all heard the adage, "Birthdays certainly beat the alternative." The same applied to my radiation treatments.

Even though I tried to find humor about the cancer growing within my body, my attitude was much more serious in the evenings when I said a prayer for all the devoted health care professionals who did everything they could to make sure I had more birthdays to celebrate in the future.

From what I have been told – to date – they succeeded. When my prostate cancer was first discovered in 2003, my PSA was 16.9 – more than four times what is considered normal. But during subsequent tests every six months since my radiation, my PSA has never exceeded 0.09.

# 5

There is nothing a smoker hates more than a former smoker who preaches constantly about the evils of tobacco.

I was once one of those smokers. I avoided former smokers almost as much as everyone in the tiny rural community of Lorena where I was born once avoided a poor man they claimed had an evil eye.

Growing up during the World War II years, every movie to appear on our small town's silver screen showed people smoking, lighting each other's cigarettes, or offering a cigarette on dates and during business discussions.

On some occasions, the smoke was so thick the film looked as if we were watching the actors through a dense fog.

The actresses were so cool in those days. During heated love scenes, beautiful women from the 1940's would put two cigarettes between ruby red lips, light them with a gold Zippo, and then with a single flourish of a snow-white arm, take one of the cigarettes and place it between the lips of their male friend, either while breathing smoke in his ear or humming three courses of "As Time Goes Bye" while sipping a martini or a favorite from "Casablanca," a champagne cocktail.

The tough guy actors were no less suave and debonair. Most of them never put a cigarette between their lips. They always held them between their upper and lower teeth to light them and then removed them with the tip of their thumb and trigger finger.

Teenagers had no choice but to smoke if they ever had any hopes of steaming the windows of a 1940 Chevy at a drive-in theater on Saturday night.

Things have changed today. It is rare to see people smoking in films, and I have become one of those former smokers who preach to my friends still addicted.

In 1990 when my pulmonary physician told me I had developed bronchial asthma and a touch of emphysema, I put my package of cigarettes in his trash can and haven't smoked since.

But I was too late.

The damage had been done after 48 years of inhaling smoke, tar, tinges of horse manure, ground up earthworms, suspected hints of urine left in tobacco fields by uncaring farm workers, and only God knows what else the cigarette manufacturers put into their products and consequently into my lungs.

My lungs were irrevocably damaged and I have had to live with the results.

The main problem?

Severe bronchitis that became a part of my life with the beginning of each winter; a problem that became worse and more difficult to heal with each passing year.

January, 2009, was the worse yet. Nothing my physician tried helped - including several different antibiotics, so many shots in my skinny behind I felt like the proverbial pin cushion, and enough steroids to make me more wired than any of the city's Christmas decorations.

On the evening of January 20, I began to cough up blood.

As you can guess, I was more fretful than I would have been had I known I was going to have to sit in a room for an hour playing bingo with a group of seniors like myself bragging about their grandchildren.

The following morning I was waiting in my physician's parking lot at 8:00 a.m. when she arrived. She immediately sent me to my pulmonary physician who set up a bronchoscopy for me the following day.

Now you haven't lived until you have experienced someone poking a tube as long as a Boa Constrictor and the size of a piece of landscape timber down your nostril; a tube made even more abrasive with a light and a camera attached to the end.

The first step in the procedure was to give me a breathing treatment, followed by spraying some foul-tasting material up my nose; both designed to deaden my nose and throat.

Half a day passed before I got over the feeling that a demented dentist had shot at least a gallon of Novocain into my mouth.

Prior to the doctor inserting the landscape timber - oops - the tube with the camera up my nose, a nurse injected a vial of magic elixir into the IV in my arm.

Before I could say, "It's not working," it worked. The next thing I knew the procedure was finished and I woke up staring into the smiling face of a friend who was by my side during the entire procedure.

I don't remember much about what happened. The only thing I do remember was my physician showing me some photographs she made of my lung; photographs that clearly showed an obstruction that looked suspiciously like a baby shucked oyster resting in a tomato sauce colored valley at the end of the bronchial tube and on top of the lung.

Once a photographer, always a photographer, I suppose, because I was almost as interested in the quality of the photographs made with such a tiny camera, as I was in hearing the results.

Of course, at the time, I was floating somewhere in the never-never-land between being stoned and pie-eyed drunk from the drugs they had given me.

Then came the difficult part.

The waiting, and waiting and waiting.

Since the procedure was done on a Friday afternoon, I did not find out the results until Monday.

As you may suspect, the two-day weekend seemed almost as long as my floor-pacing waits while my wife was in delivery rooms birthing each of my two children.

Or perhaps as long as waiting for a server who has interrupted your dinner meal at a fancy white-tablecloth restaurant several times with questions about the service; always when your mouth is stuffed, but disappears into the bowels of hell for what seems like hours while you are impatiently waiting for your check.

Or perhaps during a hard-fought football game when the score is tied and your team has one second left in the game to attempt a 55-yard field goal. The kicker moves forward, the ball is in the air, and then you wait an eternity to find out if the ball is going over the crossbar.

When my physician finally called late on Monday morning, she hesitantly told me cancer cells had been found in the biopsy.

That was when I told her, "Look, Doctor, if I have cancer cells, then let's do what is necessary to fight the little suckers."

That was also my attitude when I was told I had prostate cancer in 2004. I'm confident my positive attitude, my faith in an Almighty God, and my natural tendency to fight when I am in a situation where fighting is necessary, is what got me successfully through that ordeal.

Still, the most difficult period of waiting during my second battle with cancer was when my physician scheduled a PET Scan for me on a Friday to determine if the cancer was confined in the obstruction or if it had spread to other parts of my body.

Being a dutiful father, the first thing I did was to call my son and daughter in Texas and Minnesota to let them know the results of my bronchoscopy and to make them aware that I was set for a PET Scan on Friday.

I also warned them, "If the cancer has spread and is inoperable, I plan to spend your inheritance. For as long as I feel good, I plan to go everywhere I've always wanted to go but couldn't afford, and do the things I've always wanted to do."

They both said, in essence, "Get it on, Daddy. More power to you."

I'm sure both of them were sincere when they told me to "get it on." I'm also sure they had no idea what was going on in my mind.

Of course I'm making an assumption here, but they probably thought I would take a short cruise to the Bahamas or spend a weekend in New Orleans and then, at my age, have my fill of travel.

For sure they would not have been so cavalier had they known I was thinking about spending a week or more on the Greek island of Santorini with a dark-eyed vixen feeding me grapes.

I didn't tell them I was contemplating riding the "Alpine Express" train through the Alps in Switzerland with a companion who spoke no English but was a master communicator in Braille, or photographing mountain gorillas in Africa with Playboy bunnies serving as my camera bearers, or watching an elephant polo game in Laos where the ball was a former trainer stuffed into a gunny sack.

Neither did they know my idea of spending their inheritance meant the last check written on my account would be to the funeral home - and it would bounce.

For a man who loves to travel, I found myself - for a brief moment - no longer dreading the cancer might have spread. But only for a brief moment.

During my PET Scan, which was a cross between a CAT Scan and an MRI, the technician told me it would last around twenty minutes. When it was finally over, he helped me to my feet and said, "That wasn't too bad, was it?"

My answer to him was, "You said it would last twenty minutes. If I could make a twenty-minute love-making session appear to last that long, I would be in demand from all over the world."

The afternoon following my PET Scan, a nurse from my physician's office called with what she said was "very good news," which I later decided was both good and bad news.

The good news was the scan showed a Stage #1 cancer confined in the obstruction and no cancer anywhere else in my body.

The bad news was I had to forget about spending my kids' inheritance.

My grandiose plans to fly to Laos to watch the elephant polo games and riding the Alpine Express train in Switzerland had to be put on hold once again.

I was so thrilled at my good news from the PET Scan I spent the entire afternoon preparing dinner; a meal composed of watermelon/onion salad with raspberry vinaigrette, poached asparagus with dill dressing for an appetizer, Chicken Provencal (a Mediterranean dish in a veal Demi-glace sauce with green and black olives) and Creme Brule for dessert.

As an amateur chef specializing in Cajun and Creole cuisine, I enjoy entertaining my friends. That night was extra-special since I also wanted to share my good news with people I love and who love me in return.

I had no idea what was in store for me the following week. Only an all-knowing God was aware of what awaited me in the future. But I was not concerned that night about the future.

I had received what I considered to be excellent news, and when you are standing in a cesspool up to your nose grasping at straws, you try to grab the longest and largest straw in the pack in case you need to use it as a life preserver.

# 6

A week after I was told my PET Scan showed good news, that the cancer on top of my lung had not spread throughout my body, I met with my oncologist and the excrement hit the air conditioner.

He confirmed the cancer had indeed not spread, but he also told me my situation was not as good as I had been led to believe - or more specifically, I allowed myself to believe.

The cancer was not a small obstruction in my bronchial tube as I thought. In reality, it was a mass that touched on all three lobes in my lung.

Surgery was out of the question without removing the entire lung which would have made it impossible for me to survive, particularly with my lungs having been damaged so drastically by many years of smoking.

The news, as you may have assumed, was not just a surprise; it was a shock, especially since I had felt after the PET scan that my odds of survival were much better.

When I asked what my chances were if I did nothing, I was told in a very professional and straightforward manner I had, at the outside, four months to live.

My alternative was a regimen of chemo and radiation, which would simply, as he said, "buy me more time."

How much time was simply an educated guess.

I think the oncologist was almost as shocked as I was because I did not go into hysterics.

Perhaps it was because I had earlier prepared myself for such a diagnosis. I had long ago turned my case over to God and was willing to accept His will.

Equally as important, I remembered how my wife was told she had six months to live when her lung cancer was diagnosed, but she lived six beautiful years.

I also remembered how my brother was given less than six months with his lung cancer. That was three years ago.

Since I have always been able to keep a tight rein on my emotions when necessary, I accepted the news in a calm manner. I told my oncologist I was willing to do whatever it took to gain as much time as possible - once again, grasping at the largest straw to use as a life preserver.

Telling my son, daughter and grandson, as well as my close friends, of my diagnosis and preparing them for the fact my life span might be considerably shortened, was even more difficult than accepting the diagnosis myself.

Seeing the expressions on their faces, hearing the choking sounds in their voices, was something I had not prepared for and something I had a serious problem accepting.

Yet my children were strong as they had been taught to be from birth. They had inherited their father's ability to hide his emotions behind a smiling facade and their mother's courage and determination.

As I have already mentioned, I am a confirmed optimist. So I considered my oncology report only the first round in what I hoped would be at least a 15-rounder before I was stretched out on the canvas.

Life has not always worked as I may have wished, but those few times when I thought I had a complaint are so unimportant now I can't even remember what made me dissatisfied.

I have lived a blessed life and I thank God for every day I have lived. But I'm also a fighter. When I am put into a position where fighting is necessary, I fight with tooth and nail. There are no rules.

So I refused to believe the cancer occupying my lung was a permanent resident.

As far as I was concerned, I was like the cattle ranchers during the old west era when farmers began moving in on their range. My cancer was just a nester, a squatter, and I was arming myself for what I guessed would be a long fight.

Having to undergo radiation for eight weeks in 2004, being subjected to every kind of test available to medical science over the past four years where radiation is used, and then having to face another eight-week bout with radiation and chemo once a week, had one advantage. And this is where my imagination and weird sense of humor comes into play.

I figured I would be able to save on electricity.

I would no longer have to have night lights throughout the house. My body would glow like the pretty red-haired girl on TV who played an angel.

Neither would I have to worry about unwanted crawling and flying insects. As soon as one of them entered my house and got anywhere close to me, a blue light would flash from my body, there would be a cracking sound like one of those electronic mosquito zappers, and it would be goodbye insect.

Of course that could never happen, but it sounds good and it was the way I felt during my second bout with radiation.

Even though I was optimistic, and even though I believed with everything within me that I had a chance to beat cancer a second time, I felt better after my initial meeting with my radiologist.

He gave me hope. He gave me a reason to believe if I followed his instructions to the letter, I had a 20 to 80 percent chance. Quoting my favorite cowboy again, "Them are pretty good odds."

I knew I faced another eight weeks of daily radiation, I knew I faced the possibilities of all kinds of side effects from the radiation and the chemo, but I truly believed I would survive - and still do.

The first thing I did after I received the news that I would go through radiation again was to rush to the drug store to buy the largest package of Q-tips I could find to bathe my wrinkled old body after it had been covered again with all those black tattoos.

It was embarrassing enough to have to bathe my torso with Q-tips, but it was even more so to have to look into the mirror and see the old man's gut I swore when I was a young man I would never have. But I earned every pound of it.

I love to cook and I love to eat. And you know what? At this stage in my life I could care less.

The next thing I was told by my team of physicians was I should have a port inserted into my chest. My first questions were, "What the hell is a port, and why is it necessary to put something in my chest when my cancer is in my lung?"

Once again my imagination clicked into high gear with two scenarios.

As a man who loves cruising better than any other kind of vacation, I could picture a round, glass-covered window in my chest like the ones I had occasionally seen in some ship staterooms.

With it, I supposed, I would not have to undergo as many X-rays and CAT scans if the doctors could just pull off my shirt and look inside my body to see what was happening.

The other scenario reminded me of my 20-year tenure as Director of Public Information at Mississippi State University, and a research animal that drew attention from the media all over the United States.

Scientists had cut a hole in a cow's side and inserted a tube about three inches wide into its stomach. A plastic, removable cap protruded about an inch out of the animal's hide so it could be opened periodically and researchers could study the animal's digestive process.

My imagination was far off course in both cases. Neither of those scenarios was in store for me.

The port was a tiny round object about the size of a marble with a long tubular tail embedded into my chest under the skin with the tail inserted into a vein; looking very much like a gigantic tadpole.

With the port inserted, nothing showed from the outside, and they didn't have to stick my veins with needles the size of a large stick of pulp wood every time they gave me chemo. They simply pushed a needle through my skin into the port and the job was done.

The worst thing about having the port inserted was I had to be at the hospital at 6:30 a.m. on a Monday morning.

For a night person like me (I do most of my writing late at night), I had no idea anyone was ever awake at that time of morning, much less working and cutting on people.

Other than opening up my chest with a very thin and very sharp scalpel at a time I didn't even know the sun had risen from its long night's sleep, medical personnel do other strange things.

Almost every test I had scheduled was on a Friday at noon when normal people are sitting at a table having lunch, or in late afternoon when civilized people are sipping martinis or tall glasses of sour mash; which forced me to agonize throughout a long weekend waiting for results.

Every surgical procedure I had scheduled was performed bright and early on a Monday morning - also when I had to agonize over a long weekend, wondering if the doctor's hands would be steady after a weekend of socializing with his or her friends.

I have several physician friends so I know of what I speak. When they get just the slightest chance to get away from sick people, even for a moment, those guys and gals naturally know how to socialize.

When I asked the advantage of having a port installed, my physician said, "To keep you from being stuck with a needle every time you receive chemo. Veins soon deteriorate," and he added, unnecessarily I thought, "particularly at your age."

I asked if I couldn't go to a plastic surgeon and have a little door installed in the crook of my arm where their favorite vein is located. "That way," I said, "if they want to draw blood or insert chemo all they would have to do is open the door."

My doctor didn't crack a smile.

I realized at that moment he might have a lot of medical knowledge, but I also knew his sense of humor was not as weird as mine. But then, few people do have a sense of humor as weird as mine.

When I arrived at the hospital at 6:30 a.m., I was sleepy and grumpy as any old man forced to get out of a warm bed at 5:00 a.m. and drive to a hospital for surgery without even a cup of coffee or a bowl of prunes to start his day. I was definitely not in the mood to be greeted by happy, smiling people.

I couldn't help but remember when the news editor on a long-running TV show asked his young female reporter, "Why are you always so perky?" Then he frowned and said, "I hate perky."

Still, I reasoned if I was about to be sliced and diced, I would be better off having it done by happy people rather than by people as grumpy as me.

And sliced I was.

When I woke up following the surgery, I had two incisions in my chest about two inches long and a large lump under my skin about the size of a quail egg they said was my port.

After spending much of my life enjoying science fiction books and movies, my only hope was the lump really was what they claimed - a device to insert chemo.

Yet I couldn't erase the nagging thoughts that perhaps an evil scientist had inserted an egg from some outer space creature under my skin and was using my old body as an incubator.

I suppose I will know the answer someday if I feel pecking from the inside of my chest.

I'm sure most of you will agree that, regardless of the outcome, not knowing is many time worse than knowing.

After my initial sessions with the radiologist and oncologist, and having my port installed, I felt better and more confident.

I was certainly aware that my odds of survival were not so good I would toss the deed to my farm on the table during a poker game. But I did know the arena where my battle would be fought. I knew the weapons I would need to fight the good fight. I knew my enemy and I knew what I would have to do to defeat it.

All I had to do was maintain my courage, my positive attitude, my sense of humor and continue to believe I was in God's hands.

*"This kind of war,
you've gotta believe
in what you're
fighting for."*
*John Wayne*

# 7

During my eight weeks of radiation in 2004 for prostate cancer, I was lucky to bypass the use of chemotherapy.

So I had no first-hand knowledge about what to expect when my oncologist told me both chemo and radiation was necessary if I was going to survive, or even gain extra time, as a result of the cancer on my lung.

I had heard all kinds of horror stories about the side effects of chemo ranging from nausea to constipation, allergic rash to diarrhea, sores in my mouth to in-growing toenails, and pimples on my behind to Punxsutawney Phil seeing his shadow on Groundhog Day and forcing the nation into another six long weeks of winter.

Perhaps not exactly pimples on my behind, but those irritations were the only possibilities omitted when I was given an hour-long lecture, complete with illustrations from a loose-leaf notebook the size of the Sears-Roebuck catalog I scanned during visits as a boy to an outdoor privy, on what I might expect during my chemo treatments.

When my instructor finished explaining all that could possibly happen, I almost decided not to go through chemo.

Frankly, I was terrified.

Then I thought about my oncologist telling me, "If you do nothing, you've got a maximum of four months to live," and I quickly changed my mind.

As bad and as uncomfortable as the side effects might make me feel, nothing could be worse than what cancer could do to me if I did nothing.

The only possible side effect she outlined that did not cause concern for me was sexual dysfunction - or as my father was prone to say, the loss of my manhood.

For many men, particularly those much younger than me, I'm sure such a loss would be #1 on the list of things to cause concern. But in my case, sixteen months of hormone treatments for prostate cancer in 2004 had removed that concern semi-permanently.

Semi-permanently? What does that mean?

It means that I still can't resist looking at a perfectly formed behind, a long pair of legs and enticing cleavage.

But as a man in his early 80's filled with all sorts of alien hormones and little cancer cells with teeth the size of saber-toothed tigers gnawing on every vital they can find like a bunch of starved termites in a lumber yard, my old body no longer can keep pace with my much younger and imaginative mind.

When I first realized the hormone regimen had taken away my ability to - you know, perform - the shock was not only frustrating, it was also embarrassing.

It didn't happen slowly, giving me time to prepare. It happened instantly without me having any idea it was lurking insidiously in the wings; somewhat akin to inviting a friend home for dinner and then not being able to provide a promised home cooked meal.

Yet, despite the blow to my macho persona, I survived in much the same manner and with the same attitude as I did when my physician told me I was a borderline diabetic.

I faced the knowledge that such wonderful delicacies as chess pie, chocolate cake and butter nut ice cream were not the only pleasures I would have to give up to survive.

There was nothing left for me to do but shake my head in resignation and mutter, "*Que Sera Sera*, what will be will be." Sorry but I don't know the Spanish words (or are they Italian) for, "It's already happened and there's not a damn thing I can do about it."

Prior to my first chemo treatment, I had a week to think, imagine, sweat and prepare my mind for whatever was to come.

I imagined myself stretched out on an operating table surrounded by doctors, nurses, IV poles, and plastic tubing running in every direction except toward North Dakota or perhaps even Canada's Yukon Territory. But I was not surprised. I couldn't imagine any warm-blooded Southerner, or even plastic tubing, heading that far north unless somebody was chasing him.

I also fantasized about bags of clear liquid hanging from each of the IV poles, obviously defective bags made in Bangladesh, Japan or UCLA (Upper Corner of Lower Alabama) since they all leaked one drop at a time.

A bank of stadium quality lights suitable for night football games would naturally be suspended three feet from my face and beamed directly into my eyes, keeping me from seeing and appreciating the, shapely 25-year-old nurse attending to my medical needs.

From that point forward, I had no further basis for my imagination to work. All I knew was the chemo medication would be inserted into my body through the port physicians had previously implanted into my chest. But I couldn't figure out how they were going to accomplish their mission since a thick layer of skin covered the port.

I found the answer the hard way. But that comes later into the story.

On the morning I was to have my first treatment and reported to my oncologist's office, only two seats remained in a 50-or-more-seat waiting room. I looked at my watch. 9:50 a.m.

My appointment was for 10:00 a.m.

*All these people still here ahead of me? No way will I begin my appointment on time. No way will I begin my appointment today or even this week.*

I started to sweat, not just a damp mist, but rivulets running down the sides of my face, crossing under my neck, and forming a puddle in the crease where my gut met my chest in combat long ago and won.

Surprisingly, I waited no more than ten minutes when my name was called.

*Hey, this is not too bad. Perhaps I misjudged these people.*

Then I found out I was not to begin my chemo treatment. My call was for the inevitable blood-letting, the feeding of the leeches, the restocking of a vampire's snack bar that immediately precedes any medical procedure.

A voice from behind a door ordered me to sit down.

Minutes later a huge woman wearing a straw hat and with breasts that weighed more than I did came toward me carrying a small milking stool and a 10-gallon galvanized bucket in one hand and a large syringe with a five-inch needle on one end and a small faucet attached to the other.

She sat down on the stool in front of me, put the bucket between her knees and aimed her faucet-equipped syringe toward the crease in my elbow.

Then I opened my eyes and saw not what I had visualized, but rather an attractive nurse with a smile as broad as the Mississippi River who made me feel much better just by her touch on my arm.

As she leaned over to stick me with the needle, I could have sworn I smelled just a hint of perfume.

I knew right then I had to get control over my imagination or it would soon get control of me.

I have always been curious to know how the Red Sea got its name - and why.   But during the past six years I have had enough blood drawn from my old body to create a second Red Sea wide enough to join the Atlantic and the Pacific Oceans, as long as the Nile River, and as opaque as the muddy Mississippi.

If I could have sold all the blood taken from me, rather than paying them to take it, I would be so rich people like Bill Gates and Warren Buffet would be considered destitute.

I have, over the years, determined how much booze I can drink at a party before I start wearing a lampshade over my head.

I know I can't eat huge helpings of fried foods without having knots in my stomach the size of basketballs.

I found out almost 20 years ago it was stupid to smoke, I am too old for sex, and I have had to severely limit my intake of Tennessee's finest. But I have yet to find out how much blood can be siphoned from my old body before I run dry.

I wonder if the doctors even know the equation. When I see a sign stating, "The Practice of Medicine," I wonder what is in store for me in the future.

When the technician finished draining my blood and told me to return to the waiting room, I figured my chemo treatment would start immediately. But I was wrong. Nearly an hour later a woman with the voice of a Command Sergeant Major on steroids bellowed my name.

When I meekly followed her through the door she held open for me, the palm of her other hand pressing forcibly against my back, I wondered if I would ever return from the chemo inner-sanctum. But once again, my overly-active imagination had lured me into a pool of quicksand of its own making.

As she pulled aside a curtain for me to enter my tiny cubicle, there was no operating table, no bank of lights, and no masked doctors and nurses holding up soap-covered hands.

Instead there was a plush reclining chair, a small television set mounted to an adjustable frame, a large window facing a grove of trees welcoming Spring with its tiny green leaves, and a comfortable chair for anyone I might want to share time with me while I was hooked up to IV's.

Yet one part of the scenario I had imagined was true. Plastic tubing ran in every direction.

Although none of the tubing appeared to be leading toward North Dakota or the Yukon, I suspected most were aimed toward South Florida since the bags contained clear liquid that looked suspiciously like vodka martinis.

I thought of martinis since the photo of my cancer taken during my broncoscopy looked like a tiny raw oyster nestled into a crease on top of my lung. And as anyone with discriminating tastes knows, there is nothing better with raw oysters than a cool, crisp martini.

Yet not a one of the leaking bags had a slice of lemon or olives on a toothpick as a garnish.

When the nurse opened up my shirt to insert the chemo into the port in my chest, I asked the obvious question, "How do you get to the port since it is embedded under the skin?"

She looked at me like I was, as the old saying goes, "One brick short of a load," and held up a needle that had a strange crook at the end.

"You have a defective needle," I said. "It's bent at the end."

"Hehehehe," she laughed. "I know. It has to be that way to penetrate the skin and lock into the port so we can insert the medicine. Now stay very still," she said as she drove the strange looking needle into my port with the force of a Navy destroyer ramming an enemy submarine during World War II.

Minutes later after the maintenance staff finally pulled my head and shoulders out of the ceiling and helped me settle into my plush recliner, the nurse hooked up the first of several IV's and told me to settle back and relax.

"You will be finished in about five hours."

"Five hours?" I blurted. "Will I have to sit here five hours every week?"

"Normally you will only be here three hours," she answered. "But the first time is special. You get to watch a movie about chemotherapy."

"Can't we skip the movie," I pleaded. "I have already spent an hour hearing about all the side effects I might face. How much more frightened do you people want me to be?"

"But with the movie, it's in living color," she giggled.

*Five hours sitting alone in a tiny room smaller than my closet with no one to talk with and nothing to keep me occupied but counting drops from defective bags leaking into clear plastic tubing?*

Have you ever watched liquid falling one drop at a time?

It's like counting freight cars at a railway crossing when a train whizzes across your street - only much, much slower.

And infinitely more boring.

I knew my weird imagination had led me down a crooked road regarding the administering of chemo, but I was still floating in a never-never-land as to how my body was going to be affected with its side effects.

My nurse told me matter-of-factly as she hooked me up to the first bag of liquid, "If you're going to have an adverse reaction of any sort, it will probably happen within the first twenty-five minutes."

The effect most mentioned by people I had met who were undergoing - or had undergone - chemo was nausea, vomiting and hair loss.

Yet as the nurse left me alone in my cubicle without apparently a second thought to my possible puking potential, I saw nothing within reaching distance that would enable me to dispose of the results of nausea.

*Even commercial jet planes come equipped with barf bags.*

Not my physician's office.

There were no bags, no buckets, no potty chairs, or no bed pans. Not even a sink. But being a practical man, my eyes soon spotted a large trash receptacle located within three giant steps from my chair.

*Still, three steps can be as far as a journey into space if my nausea reacts in the same explosive manner and with the same force as a rocket does during blast off.*

Having been forewarned, for the next twenty-five minutes I sat buried up in my brown recliner twisting, squirming and sweating; waiting to find out if I would vomit, have pimples pop up on my behind, be responsible for a weird-looking groundhog causing six additional weeks of winter, or live the remainder of my life with my eyes crossed.

I had no doubt the crossed eyes would win out since I kept one eye trained on the clock counting down twenty-five minutes to see what might happen to me, and the other eye on the bag with a hole in it that kept leaking liquid out the bottom one drop at a time.

*Which might not be too bad if women feel toward cross-eyed men as I do about cross-eyed women. Nothing to me is more sexy.*

The only time my late wife ever showed any jealousy was when a cross-eyed woman appeared on television and I immediately sat straight up in my easy chair - and she immediately turned off the television set.

Despite sitting in a frozen position for twenty-five minutes waiting for the proverbial axe to fall during my first treatment, the imprints of my fingers buried into the fabric of the chair, not one adverse reaction occurred to my body from the chemo.

Neither did it occur during the third week, the sixth week nor during the final eighth week.

As far as I was concerned, I was blessed by an understanding God who was well aware of the yellow streak down my back where pain and discomfort were concerned.

The only adverse reaction I could attribute to either the radiation or the chemo was the fact I was a little more fatigued than normal - and I had a little more trouble than normal with my concentration.

When I explained my inability to concentrate to my radiation physician, he smiled and murmured, "Chemo brain."

"Chemo what?" I asked.

He smiled. "Being unable to concentrate is normal for some people after long periods of chemo. Patients who have been through it call it Chemo Brain. But just to make sure, in your situation, I'm going to make an appointment for you to have a CAT scan of your brain."

I was not pleased to undergo another CAT scan, yet I was happy my doctor was not taking anything for granted.

Two days after I had gone through the scan, I was about to receive my radiation treatment when the doctor walked up to the table and said with a slight smile, "I have good news about your scan. You have a brain."

I was so shocked to hear him show a sense of humor I sat straight up on the table, forgetting a huge machine the size of a rocket launcher was only inches away. The knot on my head from that collision was the first and only pain I endured during all my radiation treatments, both in 2004 and 2009

At least his attempt at humor served one purpose. I now had medical evidence to the contrary when my friends tell me I don't have a brain in my head.

# 8

I thought waiting over a long weekend to find the answer to a CAT scan was frustrating, but it did not compare to waiting six weeks to find out if the eight-week regimen of chemo and radiation I had just completed had any effect on my cancer.

Had its size remained the same? Had it grown? Or could it possibly have shrunk? Had my chances for an extended life improved since my original diagnosis of four months - which had thankfully passed?

These questions and many more of a similar nature continued to pester me, to gnaw at me through the many long days and nights of waiting, even though my radiologist had warned me repeatedly not to pay undue attention to the first report.

"If the report say's the cancer has not changed, that's good news. If it say's it has decreased in size that is excellent news. But even if it has grown, don't put too much credence to the report. We still have other treatments we can use before we give up the fight."

Still, each day seemed as if an additional hour had been added to the standard 24-hours we have grown to expect in a day. But as with other major events that happen in our lives, both dreaded and anticipated, the day finally rolled around when I sat across from my oncologist shaking, choking, swallowing air because there was no liquid in my mouth, and hoping against hope his long awaited prognosis was one I wanted to hear.

And it was.

All the waiting became worthwhile when he smiled and told me, "The chemo and radiation worked for you to a degree. You cancer has shrunk."

I was elated; not only because the cancer had diminished in size, but also because there was finally a shrinkage in my old body that was welcomed. But as sometimes happens with cancer and its side effects, my elation was short-lived.

For at least two weeks before my appointment, my breathing had been severely hampered. Just the slightest exertion like walking across a room or bending over to pick up something off the floor caused me to stop and gasp for breath.

My oncologist showed me a negative print of my lungs that had been taken the day before my appointment. One lung showed up as clear and black on the print, but the other was almost solid white; a problem the doctor was apparently more concerned about at the time than the cancer.

"Apparently one of your lungs was damaged to a degree by the radiation," he said, "and it is highly infected. This is a condition we will have to clear up before we can proceed with any other treatment on the cancer."

Gradually, over a three-week period, antibiotics, steroids and a steady dose of oxygen - which apparently will be my constant companion in the future - did clear up the infection to the point where I could perform my normal duties around the house and even drive and take care of my business and personal affairs.

Yet like wolves that travel in packs, side effects of cancer and cancer treatments can also raise their multiple heads at the same time like long-necked geese peeking over the tops of tall grass.

Such as puffy, swollen ankles as an accompaniment to my infected lung.

I had never been bothered with swelling joints before. So when I pulled off my shoes and saw ankles that were so swollen they looked like country hams stuffed in pillow cases, I didn't have to wear a note from my teacher pinned on my shirt to know something else was wrong.

Since I had been told that on occasions the chemo and radiation treatments can cause blood clots, both in the extremities and in the lungs, I called my doctor who immediately set me up for a Doppler scan to find out if clots were indeed in existence and if they were the cause of the swelling.

The scan showed that I did not have any clots in my large veins or arteries, but did have one in a small capillary.

Being a thorough and careful man, my oncologist put me on a regimen of shots - one a day for 14 days - to try to dissolve the clot before it possibly moved into a larger vein. At the end of the 14 days, I went through another Doppler scan which found the clot had not dissolved and had started to move. Even worse, a spot showed up on my lung the doctor firmly believed was a clot.

"What happens now?" I asked.

"We start another regimen of shots," he answered, "only stronger. And I'm also going to put you on a blood thinner."

I almost blushed when I asked him the next question because I felt stupid even saying the words. "What is the medicine you are giving me in the shots?" I laughed. "Somebody told me it was rat poison. Is that not a hoot?"

Without even the slightest smile, he said, "That's what it is. Or at least a derivative."

I almost choked. "Good Lord, Doctor, you're shooting up my body with rat poison? What does that have to do with dissolving clots? And how and when did something that dangerous become a treatment for people?"

The way he told me the story was much longer and contained many more details, but here is the gist of what he said. "Back in the early thirties, a smalltime Midwestern dairy farmer was put out of business in one night when he woke up to find all his cows were dead. They were bleeding internally, as well as from their noses, mouths and eyes.

"The farmer filled a bucket with blood from one of the cows and drove all night to the state university to have the blood analyzed in order to find out what had happened and why it had happened," he said.

"The professor he talked with was in the midst of researching ways to kill rats with more certainty than the methods used at that time. The researcher discovered the farmer's cows had been eating a certain kind of clover that had apparently caused the problem.

"From that information, he produced a compound that when ingested by the rats would cause them to bleed to death."

He smiled. "But that's not the end of the story. A doctor had read about the professor's findings and decided that given in limited doses, the compound might cause blood clots in humans to dissolve. It has been used very effectively since."

I frowned. "Is there a chance that by taking this medication I will bleed internally? Granted that in my time I've been associated with rats, even been called a rat by people with poor taste and bad judgment, but I've got enough problems without adding an on-going battle with rat poison to the list."

"No chance," he said. "We'll be giving it to you in limited strength and gradually increase the strength as needed and as your system can tolerate it. We will periodically check your blood to see how you are handling the medicine and what we should do in the future."

As I wrote in the front part of the book, I have a vivid imagination. But what I didn't write is that I am also prone to exaggerate. So I am probably making more over this "rat poison" thing that is necessary - as I did a long time ago when I was a small boy and ran home from the barn screaming to my parents about all the rats I saw.

"The minute I opened the door to the corn crib, I must have seen a thousand rats," I muttered, gasping for breath.

My father looked at me and smiled. "Now, Bob, are you sure you saw a thousand rats?"

I paused. "Well, maybe not that many. But I did see at least a hundred."

"Think again," my father said. "How many?"

I knew I was being forced to back away from what I thought was a great story, but I had no choice but to renege in the face of my father's piercing eyes and determined tone.

I sulked a second or two and said, "I know I saw at least a dozen."

Dad smiled. "That's more like it. Now tell me what you actually saw."

"Well, I did see a shuck shake," I blurted and ran out of the house.

Once an exaggerator, always an exaggerator, I suppose. I'm not sure if this has meaning, but since I have been taking the shots, every time I'm in the grocery store and pass a round of old fashioned hoop cheese, I have the strangest urge to put the entire ring in my cart. And I dread the day when my apartment manager visits my apartment and sees all the tiny holes I have gnawed in the wall.

Still, my exaggeration, combined with my active imagination, has made me a good living over the years.

Unfortunately, the blood clots in my leg and possibly in my lung - along with what happens with my cancer - must remain as unfinished parts of my ongoing saga. But I am looking at this setback with the same positive thinking and sense of humor I have been using to fight my cancer.

I am confident that in the long run, with the help of my medical staff and the blessings of God, I will also win this battle.

# 9

During the past six years while being probed, sliced and cut in hospitals and doctor's offices for prostate cancer, a coronary heart occlusion, a "rare and deadly" strain of pneumonia, and finally a cancer on top of my lung, I became painfully aware I had no say-so over what physicians did to me while searching for answers to my medical problems.

Neither did I have a say-so over the amount of time some of them made me wait over and above the hours my appointments were scheduled.

Many times while my rear end became saddle sore sitting and waiting in boring waiting rooms with nothing but outdated magazines for company, I wished some of my physicians could have been clients of mine before I retired.

In my imagination, I gloated over how much I would have enjoyed looking through a two-way mirror and watching while they squirmed and waited for me to make an appearance.

My enjoyment would have been doubled thinking the five-year-old magazines I had chosen for my physician clients to read were filled with stories about the love life of spayed boll weevils turned loose on an unsuspecting female population.

Unfortunately, that never happened – boll weevils are much too tiny for such delicate surgery, and very few doctors feel the need for public relations specialists' to repair their image.

To make time spent in a waiting room even worse - before being led to another tiny, windowless room where my only reading material was terrifying charts of my ailing anatomy - I was subjected to people who had no qualms about sharing the most intimate details of their ailments and pains, ranging from sickening to downright humorous.

During one waiting room wait, an elderly patient went into lengthy detail about the reason he was bald.

He removed his baseball-type cap and rubbed his shiny scalp as if he needed to prove his baldness.

"When I was young, I had so much hair my barber had to thin it out every time I went in for a haircut," he said. "But during my chemotherapy treatment for colon cancer, my hair came out in clumps. It kept coming out until, all of a sudden, there was no hair left to comb."

He laughed. "I have been bald ever since. What I still can't figure out is why the hair on my head came out when I was being treated for a cancer in my behind. Ain't that a hoot?"

Even though one of the most interesting people I met worked diligently to portray a character image, it took less than ten minutes for me to discover he was a highly educated and retired professional man.

Still, it took a lot of prodding for me to find out that much.

"The Good Lord created 90 percent of us as folks and ten percent of us as characters," he said with a grin.

"Without the characters, regular folks wouldn't have anything to do or to talk about. I decided many years ago I was among the ten percent."

When he offered to buy me a cold beer after we finished our appointments, I looked at my watch and shook my head. 9:20 a.m. "Too early in the morning for me."

"Never too early," he said, rousing the entire waiting room with his laughter. "I knew a man once who drank a quart of bourbon every day. But even then, it wasn't the booze that got him. He was hit by a car while walking to the liquor store."

He was fascinated when he found out I was a writer. He leaned back in his chair and proudly announced that he was also writing a book.

"I call it, *Places I Have Peed.* And when you consider all the places I have traveled, the list is long and impressive."

After I recovered from my shock at his surprising title, he explained: "I was treated for prostate cancer about 12 years ago. Then, as cancer sometime does, it came back. Now, I am being treated with a series of hormone shots - along with the radiation - that seem to be working. So you see, bathroom visits are one of the most important functions in my life."

During an appointment with another physician, I sneezed loudly while reading a magazine where a wordy writer had taken three pages to describe how Angelina Jolie became pregnant with twins (I could have said the same thing with three words).

A man next to me asked, without prior chit-chat, "Have you ever had allergy shots?"

"Yes," I mumbled, thinking more at the time about Angelina Jolie's twins being conceived than my allergies.

"The shots really worked for me," he said. "I just wish my regular doctor could be as good at finding a way to cure my hemorrhoids."

Thank goodness my name was called before he went into detail describing his treatment.

Let's face facts, folks. Thinking of Angelina Jolie and hemorrhoids at the same time is not a pleasurable sensation.

On another occasion, a somewhat obese woman enlightened us about her chest infection.

She described her coughing in such living color those of us who were only waiting for regular check-ups became so ill we stood in line to get into the bathroom.

While waiting one morning to have the surgical procedure to put a port in my chest, I met this older gentleman (a World War II vet) who was waiting to have surgery to remove a cancer from his nose.

"The first thing I asked my doctor," he said with a grin, "was if I could still smell food. I've always had a good nose, but nothing like my wife." He laughed. "She has such a good sense of smell I could use her to hunt rabbits or squirrels. I tease her by calling her my beagle with two legs."

Many years ago, before either of my battles with cancer, I had the opportunity for a long chat with a middle-aged man who not only declared he was homeless, but also bragged that he had been a bum for more than 30 years.

His ragged jeans and long-sleeved shirt looked as if they had not been washed or even removed in weeks. He wore a baseball cap and a long, unkempt beard.

Since he chose to sit in the chair beside me, and being a journalist and a curious man, I took advantage of the opportunity to visit with him - even though I had to breathe through my mouth every time I turned my face toward him.

After we had talked for about five minutes, he said, "Sir, I haven't eaten in two days. Would you have enough change for me to buy some food when I leave here?"

Being a cynical man, I assumed if I gave him money, he would spend it on beer or wine rather than food. But there was something about him that made me change my mind. I handed him a $5 bill with the stipulation that he answer some questions for me.

After he snatched the bill out of my hand and stuffed it into his shirt pocket, he asked, "What do you want to talk about?

"You," I said. "I'm a writer and . . . ."

He laughed. "And you want my long, sad story, how I was mistreated as a child, got hooked on booze and dope, and lost my job, wife and children. Right?"

"Is that the way it was?"

He laughed again. "Not even close, friend. My parents were fine people who did everything they could to raise me right and to give me a start in life. Even though I might enjoy a good, cold beer on a hot day, or even a shot of bourbon when there is a chill in the air, I am neither a drunk nor a doper."

"Then why. . . .?"

"Why am I sitting here in dirty clothes begging for money from a perfect stranger?"

"Something like that," I said.

"Because some people are destined to be bums from the day they are born and there's not a thing all the religious zealots or psychologists in the world can do to prevent it."

"You sound like an educated man."

"Would you believe I had two years of college?" he asked. "But one night while I was cramming for an exam, I realized that for me, life had to be more than working and paying taxes. I threw my book across the room, packed my toothbrush, a clean shirt, some socks and underwear in a bag and walked out the door. That was more than thirty years ago."

He paused. "Are you by any chance driving the big pickup in the parking lot with the fifth-wheel trailer hitch in the bed?"

"Yes," I smiled.

"Then you and I are not that different."

I frowned. "Are you saying I am a hobo?"

He laughed. "I haven't heard that word in years. You're telling your age, you know."

"Why did you say we are not that different?"

"You are just a wealthier and more sophisticated bum. You have a trailer that you pull behind your truck? Right?"

I nodded.

"You have obviously worked hard, saved your money and invested it carefully so you could buy your truck and trailer and travel around the country without someone giving you orders."

When I did not answer, he said, "See what I mean? The difference between us is that I began enjoying my freedom a long time ago, and you wasted a lot of good years punching a clock."

I didn't look at him, not wanting him to know how correct he had been. Then on impulse, I handed him another $5 bill.

"For better days," I said.

He started to wave the money away, but changed his mind and quickly plucked the bill out of my hand. He acknowledged me with a sad smile. "As you said, friend, for better days."

During an early morning visit, only two people were in the waiting room when I arrived. A man that appeared to be somewhere in his seventies and a younger woman who had obviously lost her hair and wore a stocking cap over her head.

After she was called for her radiation treatment, I asked him, "Was that your wife?"

He laughed. "Thank you for the compliment. That lady is my daughter. My wife died after we spent 58 years together."

Although he stared several minutes at the parade of people entering and leaving the room, he really didn't see them. All he saw was the past.

"My wife died in church." he said, his voice almost gentle." She had a bad heart. The doctor told us to prepare, that death could come any second. On the morning it happened, a cold rain had been falling all night. After breakfast, when we normally began getting ready for church, I suggested that we stay at home with the weather being so bad. But she wouldn't hear of it. 'I've got your clothes already laid out and we're going to preaching as we always have," she said."

I waited silently.

"We belonged, still belong for that matter, to a little country church with a small congregation. But that morning, the morning she died, we had the biggest crowd I had seen in a long time. In fact, I even counted the people. It was 114, as I recollect.

"My wife saw what I was doing and asked, 'How many?' When I told her, she said, "It's good there's such a big crowd here today.' The second the spoke the words," he paused to snap his fingers, "she was gone just that quick."

He rubbed his eyes, stood and stretched his back when his daughter returned. As they started to leave, I said, "You didn't tell me your name?

"My name is Henry, but my friends call me Buster," he answered. He was about to close the front door behind him when he turned toward me and said, "You can call me Buster."

I have wondered many times why people, when they are told a person has been diagnosed with cancer, can't just say they are sorry, offer to help if there is anything they can do, and perhaps put the person's name on their prayer list.

What do the majority of people do? The one thing they should not do to a cancer patient. They instantly go into long-winded stories about one of their relatives or friends - and I hate this expression - that is or was "eaten up with cancer."

Every time I hear that expression my imagination conjures up a picture, such as we occasionally see on the Nature Channel, of some poor animal that has mistakenly waded into a stream and is attacked by thousands of piranhas that strip it down to the bones in a matter of minutes.

People who spread their gory stories feel it is their duty to tell a newly diagnosed person, who is already in a state of fear, all the frightening details.

Before I was diagnosed with the cancer on my lung, I had heard people talking in such a manner to cancer patients.

At the time I wished I either had the nerve to pop them in the mouth with a good right hook, or else that I had a gym sock (preferably one that had been used) to stuff into their mouths.

Now that I'm on the other side of the cancer prognosis, I probably won't do either. But one thing I can and will do is to walk away leaving them talking to themselves.

Or perhaps I will simply say, "Sir or madam," as the case may be, "my own mind is creating enough frightening scenarios without hearing your story of gloom and doom. So may we please change the subject?"

The way I view my situation, there has to be a good side to having a cancer in my lung.

As I told my minister and his wife during a delightful lunch after church services, "I no longer have to diet, and I no longer have to sip a glass of wine during 5:00 o'clock tea time rather than to enjoy my glass of Tennessee sour mash that I gave up more than two years before.

"I no longer have to put up with people who are boors," I continued, "I no longer have to take crap from anybody. And probably best of all, I no longer have to be politically correct."

Another good side of having lung problems, and having to carry a portable oxygen bottle slung over my shoulder everywhere I go, is being able to ride in carts when I go shopping at Sam's Club, Walmart or one of the large grocery stores.

When my physician first put me on oxygen, I was embarrassed. I felt I was too macho to allow my friends to see me with one of those straps in my nose and riding in one of those "old people's carts."

Yet, after a persuasive friend insisted I at least try, I discovered a new world. All of a sudden, I became Tony Stewart roaring around a track - driving only to the left, of course - and bowling over shoppers like he would other cars during a crowded race.

I was even tempted to carry a can of spray paint to write my sponsor's name on the side of the cart like other famous drivers..

My only problem was I didn't have a sponsor.

The only people I have been associated with over the past six months have been physicians and hospital personnel.

Yet I'm not sure how the leadership of St. Dominic Health Services would feel seeing the name of their Cancer Center emblazoned in bright red on the side of a grocery cart - particularly a cart driven by a wild and crazy man who might be sending them an ongoing line of mangled and battered shoppers.

No one was safe as I careened through the aisles, around the shirt racks, through the shoe shelves, down the grocery aisles, smashing through the hardware department, slowing for a danger flag while passing through ladies lingerie, and finally to the exit door where an ancient retiree with more muscles than a 103-year-old man should have, collared me and forced me to leave my vehicle in their parking garage.

I looked at him and smiled - no, I smirked. "Give it a good once over in the shop tonight. I'll be back tomorrow."

As I turned my back and ambled out of the store, I could have sworn I heard the sounds of gunshots reverberating from the front office.

Another thing I have wondered about is why people who are so private they refuse to divulge their salaries or their age, will bore you for hours about a minor ailment that could be cured with a couple of aspirin.

If I knew the answer to that question, I would be a wealthy oncologist or radiologist - with a waiting room overflowing with talkative patients rather than a hard-working writer sitting by myself in a darkened room staring at a computer monitor.

*"Well, there are some things a man just can't run away from."*
*John Wayne*

# 10

**M**any years ago when my father was in his seventies, he was diagnosed with prostate cancer. During his era, men simply did not go to doctors for exams as most do today. It was not considered a manly thing to do.

During all the time he was being treated, he never called his *prostate* anything but a *prostrate*. For many years I didn't know the difference. Until I realized I had to be *prostrate* for my doctor to examine my *prostate*. My doctor also corrected me when he sent me to a urologist.

"At least learn to pronounce your body part correctly," he said with a grin. "I would be embarrassed for my urologist friend to know I had a patient who not only had an abnormally large prostate, but an abnormally small vocabulary."

Then he smiled as he stuck his hand out, not to shake hands but to retrieve my check.

My father's urologist made the decision, as mine did when my prostate cancer was diagnosed, not to correct the problem with surgery but rather to treat him with hormones.

He had been on the regimen only a short time when he broke out in a rash that caused him to scratch so violently, particularly during his sleep, he woke up with blood all over his sheets.

When he made an appointment with his physician, he was told that the only way his life could be saved was to remove his testicles.

My father was a virile man, a highly sexual man, so he had to do a lot of what he called "Baptist meditating" before he would give the doctor an answer.

Yet he was also humble and a well-loved man. Perhaps the reason was because he never felt his importance. He never boasted about his accomplishments, never put himself into the forefront of programs in which he was involved. He simply went about his life gaining friends and respect for the man of inner strength his family and friends knew and loved.

Twice in his life, I played a small role in seeing his ego massaged. Twice in his life I was there to see him actually – well, strutting - with his feeling of importance and I could not have been more pleased.

The first time was when I was Director of Public Information at Mississippi State University. I had made arrangements with a large, international oil company for a helicopter to take me to one of their offshore drilling rigs. I was scheduled to interview the engineer in charge for a story to be published in the University's alumni magazine.

Since my father and I rarely had time to spend quality time together, I invited him to ride with me.

On our long drive to south Louisiana, he reiterated something I had heard from him most of my life: "Nothing will ever get me up in an airplane." But after mulling over my upcoming helicopter flight, he finally admitted he would like to see what it would feel like to leave the ground.

"Only if we will go no higher than ten feet," he added. "That will be high enough for me to get the feeling I want."

When we arrived at the helicopter landing pad, and I told the pilot about my father's desire, I changed the rules. "Put him in the front seat beside you and I'll sit in the back. Once you are airborne," I said, laughing, "if he doesn't have a stroke, just keep going."

The helicopter we were to use was small. The front was simply a glass bubble that made a front seat passenger feel as if there was nothing under him but space.

I could tell Dad was nervous, but he tried not to show it to the pilot – until the helicopter kept rising higher and higher and finally moved forward at a rapid clip over the beautiful Louisiana marshland.

Rather than sitting white-knuckled in fear as I had anticipated, Dad laughed and leaned forward for a better look. "Thank you, son," he said almost in reverence, "this is so beautiful."

The only time I noticed any fear in his voice or in his body language was when we arrived at the drilling rig and the pilot pointed at the landing pad that from our height looked about the size of a postage stamp.

After we landed, our pilot, who obviously had somewhat of a sick sense of humor, told the rig manager - without mine or my father's knowledge – that Dad was a senior vice president for the company who was visiting incognito for a private look at how his rig was operating.

From that moment on, we were treated like royalty, including Dad wearing a new company hard hat they presented to him as a gift with his name stenciled across the front.

On our 50-mile flight back to shore, I sat in front with the pilot who instructed me to put on a pair of earphones so we could converse without Dad hearing. That was when he told me about the joke he had played on his friends at the rigs.

When we landed, still wearing his new logo-emblazoned hard hat, Dad said, "The flight was like nothing I had ever imagined. It was like sitting on a magic carpet. And, I'll tell you something else," he added. "I've never been treated so well in all my life. I felt like a dignitary, like I was somebody really important."

I glanced at the pilot and mouthed the words, "Thank you."

The next time I witnessed Dad feeling his importance was when I served as a Senior Vice President for Blue Cross Blue Shield of Mississippi.

Dad came to the facility one day to work out a problem with a claim. After he finished, he visited with me in the executive building.

Since he had never seen the entire complex, I took him on a guided tour. As we entered each of the many departments, employees looked toward me and spoke. "Good morning, Mr. Moulder."

I noticed when I returned their greetings, Dad respond as well with more than his normal friendliness.

When our tour was over and we returned to my office, Dad looked at me and said, "You know, Bob, I had no idea how many people out here knew me."

Since he had no conception the employees could possibly be speaking to his son rather than to him, I bit my lip to keep from smiling. "You've just got a lot of friends, Dad."

When he finally came to the conclusion that he had lived an exciting life where the opposite sex was concerned, and if losing what he called his "manhood" was the only way to save his life, he had no choice but to agree.

"Besides," he told me, "I'm almost eighty and there is not much left for me anyway where the ladies are concerned."

He agreed to the surgery and all went well for several years. Then one night, only weeks before he died, the man I had never heard say one word against God and His overall plan for the human race, said, "You know, son, I've decided there is only one thing wrong with God's plan for men."

For a moment I was numb. I couldn't imagine Dad saying something against God. "What would that be?" I asked.

"I think when a man gets to be eighty years old, it would be a lot better if God took your manhood and let you keep your teeth."

My mother was not as fortunate.

After she went through surgery for what her physicians declared to be an inoperable tumor spread throughout her brain like tiny streams, she lived four months; but she never spoke again. During her last month, she did not recognize me, my brother or any of her friends.

With one exception.

Mother and my daughter, Patti, had a special relationship, as did my father and my son, David. When Patti was graduated from the University of Southern Mississippi and received her commission as an Army Lieutenant, and later finished her training as a helicopter pilot at Fort Rucker, Alabama, she received orders to be stationed in Germany.

Before she left, Mother hugged her and promised she would still be alive to welcome her home after her tour. Perhaps it was coincidence or perhaps it was God's will, but Patti returned home a few days before Mother died.

The first thing she did was to go to the nursing home to see Mother. To my surprise and to the shock of her nurses, the moment Patti entered the room, Mother's eyes widened, she smiled and held up both arms welcoming her for a hug.

Perhaps it is because Patti and I want to believe, but both of us feel confident Mother knew Patti was on her way home and waited for her as promised before she gave in to the angel of death. Her welcome was a memory neither Patti nor I will ever forget.

With both of my parents and my wife dying as a result of cancer, I wondered what else the disease would do to our family.

Then I received a call from my younger brother. His physicians had found a large cancer in his lung, so large it was stuck to the lining of his heart so surgery was prohibitive.

He, too, was projected to have a short life - six months to be exact. But his physicians put him on a regimen of chemo and radiation and after three months, they gave him the good news the cancer was shrinking. That was three years ago.

His experience and my wife's experience, of being told they had less than six months to live, is what gives me hope.

Perhaps it won't be the same for me, but as long as I have a breath in this old body, the glass is not only half full, it is running over the edge. But that is the only way I know how to think and to live.

# 11

When my wife was going through her six-year bout with lung cancer - chemo, radiation and surgical procedures in both lungs - I never understood why she was always smiling, why she was invariably in a good mood (except when I did something stupid) and why she never *po-mouthed* as we southerners are prone to say when someone is a whiner.

When I finally asked the question to her, she said, ""Because I have a positive attitude. I try to look at what I'm doing with a sense of humor, and primarily because I have put my faith in God and I believe He will take care of me."

While I was in college, if I had majored in *Faith, Attitude and Humor,* I would have had to go through four years of instruction to learn what she said in those few words.

The things she taught me when she knew she was going to die, helped me to survive my first battle with cancer and made it possible for me to endure what possibly could be my last battle.

During my last days and weeks and months of radiation and chemo, I talked to dozens of people about the value of faith, attitude and a sense of humor to the healing process. I talked to patients, therapists, physicians, ministers and cancer survivors.

Each person I talked with had a different opinion, expressed their feelings with different words, and was affected in different ways. But the end result was, "Through my faith, my sense of humor and a positive attitude, I am a winner. I am a survivor."

My son, David, who lives in Minnesota, a true believer and a former army helicopter gunship pilot who refers to himself as a warrior for his country and a warrior for God, said, "It is said darkness is the absence of light. Then wouldn't it stand to reason that sadness is the absence of joy?

"The bible describes Heaven as a place full of light and joy without sickness or pain," he continued. "God asks us to come to Him for comfort and peace. He say's He will be our 'Strong Tower', our 'Fortress,' our 'Comforter,' and He is 'the truth and the life.' Only joy can survive in His presence.

"So here is a prescription," he continued. "Turn and walk into His light. Be filled with the joy of the Lord. Filled until your cup has run over. Filled so there is no more suffering and no more pain. Filled so joy will overflow to others who so desperately need it. And then you will know a joy that outshines all things."

Bill Buckley, my son's dear friend from the first grade until the present, a former standout wide receiver at Mississippi State University, drafted by the New York Jets, and now a campus director at Mississippi College for the Fellowship of Christian Athletes, told me a story that, more than most, exemplified the power of a positive attitude.

"'We ain't losin'. Run it behind me.' Those words were spoken by Trey Hopson, Gulf Coast Community College football player, with 8:30 left in the 4th quarter in a battle of two unbeaten teams," Bill said. "Jones County Community College was the foe with everything at stake for both teams.

"Gulf Coast was ranked 3rd nationally and Jones 4th. Whoever won would not only win the Mississippi state title but would play for the national championship. That game was like a raging forest fire from start to finish. Seconds before Trey Hobson declared victory, head coach Steve Campbell gathered his offensive unit around him on the sidelines. He told them, 'Guys, we hold the ball on this drive, we win.' Gulf Coast was up 20-16 and none of us present could remember a football team holding the ball on a sustained drive for eight minutes.

"That was when 5'11", 240-pound blocking back Trey Hobson stepped up. 'We ain't losin'. Run it behind me.' I love what that statement said about Trey. He didn't say, 'Give me the ball and let me be the star.' He modeled for all of us the kind of attitude necessary for a servant-leader. He took responsibility for the fight and did it in a way that put others in front of himself. He was willing to do the dirty work and get no credit.

"What if every young husband told his wife in the heat of the battles of marriage, 'Sweetheart, I'm in this for life. We ain't losin. Run it behind me.' What if every Daddy in America told his kids, 'You can count on me to be here through thick and thin. We ain't losin.' Run it behind me.' What if every Christian promised God, 'I'll be whatever you want me to be and do whatever you want me to do. We ain't losin.' Run it behind me, Lord."

"That kind of attitude would change the face of the church and America. Well, Gulf Coast did hold the ball on that final drive for about eight full minutes and won the game. They went on to go undefeated and win the national championship as well. There is no way they could have done it without Trey Hopson, an undersized guy with an over-sized heart and the right attitude."

My minister and dear friend, the Reverend Robert C. Lane, pastor of the First Presbyterian Church in Madison, Mississippi, said, "Why do I believe a positive attitude is important? Not because a positive attitude has the power to change circumstances, but because our positive attitude is a reflection of our faith in God who is able to change circumstances.

"Our focus should never be upon our thoughts and attitudes, which directs everything inward, but upon the grace, majesty, love, mercy, compassion, power and awesome greatness of God which turns everything away from us to focus on Him.

"We can change nothing," he added, "but we worship a God who rules and over-rules all things. A positive attitude will not make us one bit healthier than we were, but it reflects our faith and trust in God who loves and cares for his children.

"A positive attitude will not effect change, but it is a statement of faith that is able to effect change. The emphasis must be removed from us and our inner being and must be turned toward God."

Finding cancer survivors with positive attitudes is like going on an Easter Egg Hunt - you never know where someone will turn up to give you a boost when you may be "back-sluding," as one of Mississippi's favorite sons, Dizzy Dean, was quoted once during an interview.

I found such a person quite by accident when I went to the Community Bank in Jackson to conduct a financial transaction. Her name? Ethel Watson.

She is a vice-president and a charmer with a smile that lights up a room. She may never realize what she did for me that day. But in a few words, she did more to boost my self confidence than most people do in an entire conversation.

She has a cancer in her lung, has gone through months of radiation, and her last treatment was with cyber-knife radiation. But she was still at work, still confident and still smiling.

"I vowed to beat this thing from the first moment I was told I had cancer," she said in a fiesty tone. "I have been treated off an on for three years and I'm still here. And I'm going to continue to be here. I believe I'm going to survive, so I refuse to allow negative thoughts to enter my mind."

*"All battles are fought by scared men who'd rather be some place else."*
John Wayne

# 12

Throughout both of my bouts with cancer, I have tried to remain positive, to retain my sense of humor, and to lean on my faith. Those things are what I am continuing to do, and what I will be doing as long as I have a breath in my body.

Yet no matter how strong a person's will may be, no matter how positive he or she may be, and no matter how strong his or her faith in an Almighty God may be, there are days when doubts creep into that person's psyche.

There are days when a person needs to escape, to find freedom from the pain and fear and negativity that takes control on his or her thinking.

A day like that happened to me not long after I finished my eight weeks of chemo and radiation and was undergoing a six-week waiting period until I could find out if my treatment had made any noticeable difference in the cancer occupying my body.

Not being a person who can sit alone and feel sorry for himself, I did something I had not done in more years than I can remember - I went on a picnic all by myself.

I bought a bucket of fried chicken wings, a fat country biscuit, a bottle of water, and drove up the famed Natchez Trace Parkway to a picnic spot on the Pearl River called River Bend where I sat at a sun-bathed table overlooking the river and meditated on my life and what was I was going through during my so-called twilight years.

With the exception of one old man fishing in the shallows about 200 yards away, no one else was around to interfere with my solitude. And even he was not breaking the silence with a noisy motor.

He used a short oar from the front of his small aluminum boat to slowly scull from stump to stump in search of a quarry that never answered his call.

The entire time I sat at my table enjoying my lunch and watching his slow and deliberate movements – which from the distance appeared almost like slow motion - he didn't catch a fish.

I didn't care.

I don't think he did either.

We were just two contented souls enjoying nature as it was meant to be enjoyed, quietly, undisturbed by worldly sounds, and with a great deal of reverence.

The noon sun was warm on my back.

The wind was still.

Not a needle stirred in the tops of the tall pine trees.

Without a ripple to mar its surface, the river looked like a pane of opaque yellow glass.

A Great Blue Heron, standing like a statue on a submerged log, waited with unlimited patience for a meal to swim its way. A fat gray squirrel, holding a hickory nut in its mouth, ran across the paved driveway toward its nest somewhere in the forest.

An alligator about eight feet long, swam slowly through a path of lily pads and climbed laboriously onto a log where it stretched out to enjoy the warm noon sun.

The line of turtles that had been using the log as a resting place, quickly moved on to a safer location.

A line of large black ants scurried back and forth across one end of the table, carrying tiny crumbs from a piece of bread someone before me had left on the table.

I didn't bother them and they didn't bother me.

It was that kind of "make love, not war," day.

Other than the raucous calls provided by five agitated crows flitting from tree to tree, I heard no other sounds. But I knew I was not alone.

I felt confident I had been guided by a power greater than myself to come to that particular place at that particular time. And I no longer felt the negative thoughts that had crept into my mind. I felt alive, confident and thankful for all my many blessings.

It was almost as if I were being directed, not only to look deeply within my inner being for humility and an understanding my life was not mine to control alone, but also to offer thanks for the wonderful life I had enjoyed for more than three-quarters of a century.

I thought of many things while I watched nature's wonders unfolding before me.

I thought how fortunate I was, while playing the starring role in the third act of my life, to be facing the future with enthusiasm, despite the obvious dangers that possibly may await me in the future.

Most importantly, I thought about the best gift I had received - the beauty and wonder of life.

After being diagnosed with prostate cancer in 2004 and lung cancer in 2009, I thought how easily it would have been to retreat into a shell and await the inevitable outcome usually associated with cancer.

But I didn't.

I refused to give in to my fears, refused to feel sorry for myself, and refused to stop living my life as an adventure as I had always done.

I thought of all these things while sitting on a hard bench, feeling a warm sun on my back, and watching the mighty Pearl River flow unimpeded toward the Gulf Coast.

I thought about other things as well – the love of my family, a multitude of friends who are always there for me as I am for them, and the God-given talents I was given at birth – talents that give purpose to my life.

A few weeks later, I had my six-week meeting with my oncologist and received what I considered to be both good and bad news.

The good news was, as my doctor told me with a broad smile, "The combination chemo and radiation treatments you have received have obviously worked to a degree. Your cancer has shrunk. In fact, you are doing so well I'm not even going to put you through additional chemo at this time. We'll just keep a close watch and see what happens."

The bad news was one of my lungs not only was damaged to some degree by the radiation, but it also was highly infected from a bout with bronchitis; making it difficult for me to breathe without supplementary oxygen and occasional bouts of antibiotics and steroids.

When I asked my physician if the condition was permanent, she answered, "We can eliminate the infection, and there is a possibility, although doubtful, the lung will improve over time. But whether or not that happens is in God's hands rather than in mine."

I smiled and silently repeated the prayer I had made in 2004 when diagnosed with prostate cancer, in 2009 with my new diagnosis of lung cancer, and many times in between:

"God I'm placing myself in your hands. This does not mean I'm not going to fight this insidious parasite for as long as I have the strength, in every avenue open to me. But after all is said and done, what happens to me is Your choice, Your plan, and I'll accept Your verdict."

# Epilog

I remember vividly sitting on a hard classroom chair at the University of Southern Mississippi and listening to my journalism professor droning on and on about how important lead paragraphs and ending paragraphs are to stories.

His opinion was the lead paragraph in a story should hook the reader and make him or her want to read more. But both he and I believed just as strongly, perhaps more so in my case, that the last paragraph should make readers smile, or cry, or feel some other equally strong emotion; should make readers happy they took the time out of their busy lives to read the story.

I write about endings because, unfortunately at this time, my story has no ending. I have no idea what is in store for me in the future.

As my oncologist told me, "I'm going to be blunt. You have a cancer in your lung and cancer has a way of doing pretty much what it wants to do, despite all we physicians can do to keep it under control."

Even as he talked, I remembered a large sign I saw a long time ago in a science laboratory at Purdue University:

***Even under the strictest scientific circumstances, bacteria do what they damn well please.***"

The doctor continued by saying, "So the odds are your health will gradually deteriorate. But if it doesn't, we'll all pat ourselves on the back and shout hallelujah."

I don't know if I will still be alive when you read this book. Only God, in His infinite wisdom, has the answer to that question. But whatever is in store for me, I am ready.

To those of you who have cancer, or who are the primary caretakers for loved ones with cancer, I hope my book has given you a reason to smile, a reason to hope, and a reason to believe.

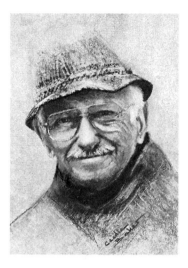

# **About the Author**

Bob Vance Moulder is a Mississippian by birth, a Southerner by preference, an American by the Grace of God, a writer by temperament, a vagabond by choice, and a confirmed optimist because he has never known another way to live.